Anxiety In Relationship

An Easy-To-Follow Guide On How To Avoid Jealousy, Conflicts, And Negative Thoughts By Improving Couple Communication Skills, Habits, And Intimacy For A Better Relationship

John Myers

&

Ashley Anita Gray

Copyright - 2021 - All rights reserved.

The content contained within this book may not be reproduced, duplicated or transmitted without direct written permission from the author or the publisher.

Under no circumstances will any blame or legal responsibility be held against the publisher, or author, for any damages, reparation, or monetary loss due to the information contained within this book. Either directly or indirectly.

Legal Notice:

This book is copyright protected. This book is only for personal use. You cannot amend, distribute, sell, use, quote or paraphrase any part, or the content within this book, without the consent of the author or publisher.

Disclaimer Notice:

Please note the information contained within this document is for educational and entertainment purposes only. All effort has been executed to present accurate, up to date, and reliable, complete information. No warranties of any kind are declared or implied. Readers acknowledge that the author is not engaging in the rendering of legal, financial, medical or professional advice. The content within this book has been derived from various sources. Please consult a licensed professional before attempting any techniques outlined in this book.

By reading this document, the reader agrees that under no circumstances is the author responsible for any losses, direct or indirect, which are incurred as a result of the use of information contained within this document, including, but not limited to, - errors, omissions, or inaccuracies.

TABLE OF CONTENTS

INTRODUCTION 10

CHAPTER 1 - How to Understand Each Other in the Relationship and Stop Fighting Constantly................................ 12
Practices for Support 13
Show Empathy More.. 14
Be More Forgiving 16
How to Know if Your Relationship Is Really Worth It? 17
Consult a Professional... 22

CHAPTER 2 - How to Decode Cryptic Messages? 24
Being a Better Listener 25
Ask More Questions 26
Practice Active Listening 26
Wait Before Responding 27
Take Note of the Tone 27
Take Note of the Modifying Words 28
Take a Holistic View 29
Follow Where the Line Leads 30

CHAPTER 3 - How to Stop Blaming or Insulting Each Other, Making Accusations, Losing Control of One's Emotions, Sometimes Starting to.. 34
Know the Other Person's Perspective... 36
Control Your Verbal and Non-Verbal Body Language 37
Construct Your Sentences as Opinions and Not Facts............. 38
Do Not Take Disagreements Personally 39

Tips for Diffusing Arguments with Your Partner 40
Pick Your Battles 40
Calm Down 41
Stick Only to the Topic 42
Watch Your Body Language, Tone, and Mannerisms 43
Accept Your Differences 44

CHAPTER 4 - Managing Problems and Negotiating Solutions 46
What's the Difference in Negotiation and Compromise? 46
Why Both Are Needed Skills in a Successful Relationship 47
Compromise Should Involve Both Sides Giving to Meet in the Middle 48
Negotiation Is a Higher-Level Way to Get What You Both Want 49
Never Discuss Compromise or Negotiation When Angry 49
Involve a Mediator if You Get Stuck 50

CHAPTER 5 - Insecurity 52
Symptoms of Insecurity and How to Recognize Them 52
Blaming 52
Playing the Victim 53
Being Jealous 54
Fearing Rejection 54
Always Having the Last Word 55

CHAPTER 6 - Spiritual Healing Techniques 62
How to Regain Your Partner's Trust 64
Love and Long-term Relationship 66

CHAPTER 7 - How To Stop Negative Thinking In Your Relationship 70
Are We Both Willing to Change Our Habits? 70

How Do We Work Together to Strengthen Our Relationship? 72

Where Are We Headed as a Couple? Where Will We Be in 5 Years? 74

What Now? 77

CHAPTER 8 - Moving on With Your Life 80
Rebuilding Your Self-Confidence 82

Stay away from negativity and negative people 82

Develop a Positive Attitude. 83

Accept Failure 83

Accept Compliments 84

Compliment Yourself 84

Do Not Compare Yourself to Others 85

Let Go of The Past 85

Practice Good Self-care 86

Believe in Yourself 86

Learning to Love Again 87

Try and visualize yourself in a new relationship that meets all of your needs 88

Do not let Fear of Ending up in Another Codependent Relationship Put You Off 89

Define Boundaries from the Start 89

Be Open to New People. 89

CHAPTER 9 - Getting to Know the True You: Being Your Authentic Self 90
Do You Know Your True Value? 90
Reasons Why You Are Unique 90
Building an Unbeatable Self Confidence That Will Always Defeat Jealousy 93
.... 93
CONCLUSION 100

INTRODUCTION

Thank you very much for purchasing this book.

Immature love loves someone for what they do well; mature love loves someone despite what they are doing wrong.

Simple couples therapy is designed to access accessible therapy and does not require careful thought or understanding (something most people find too difficult to use and apply) to be useful. On the other hand, they are not couples who are stupid enough to deny them when they need help or too guilty to fight them when they give it to them. Nor is it for newly trained therapists who feel they need to listen and indulge in the needless and unnecessary fear of not disturbing their clients. It is not for couples where, instead of trying to strengthen and improve their relationship, each couple must be right and find their own way. It's common for people to want to be honest, find their own way, and be disappointed when they don't. It is also natural that some people are right and find a way to get angry when they don't.

Each of them can be tolerated, talked about and even overcome. However, whenever one of the partners has to be right and find their way, something threatening or wrong, or if they can't find their way, they will be seen as an attack and will do everything they can to defend their position by resisting and reacting.

The goal of therapy is to train each partner to respond to the inevitable disagreements, disappointments, anxieties and frustrations in their relationship by not being upset or angry, or by excluding or avoiding each other. Enjoy.

CHAPTER 1 - How to Understand Each Other in the Relationship and Stop Fighting Constantly

Ups and downs are part of the relationship. Where there is love, there are conflicts, disagreement, and miscommunication as well. To minimize such events, try to avoid conflicts and do
everything to gain your partner's love and attention.
By doing so, you tend to bottle up your feelings and needs.

In this process, the bottle becomes full, and you realize that you are the only one in your relationship, which is putting all the efforts to make the link right. When you feel alone and taken for granted, you will experience the hurt and tend to feel angry with your partner. This pattern will lead to more adverse circumstances and cannot make you happy. There is a better way for you to adopt.

With the help of compassionate self-awareness, you will tolerate your emotions and learn to value yourself. You will become a positive person and will be able to take positive feedback from the caring and loving people in your life.
Consequently, you will be able to ignore the negative energy and will focus on the positive aspects of the relationship. It will help to maintain an intimate

relationship with your partner. When you are expressive positively and enjoyably, then healthy relationships are maintained. You will be able to know the coping mechanism to deal with the conflicts you face in the relationship.

Practices for Support

Asking for support is the approach that helps to nurture the relationship. Asking what you want and need in a relationship helps to make the relationship stronger. Two basic practices help in this matter.

Always share your wants, needs, and feelings with your partner. Sharing thoughts makes both of you understand each other better. Ask concretely and directly to your partner what you need and want from them.

Sharing your thoughts and speculations with your partner is always a good idea. You both should know what you both are going through. When you both think and reason each other, you both will be on the same page, and resolve issues will be more comfortable.

If you do not like anything about your partner, it is best to tell him rather than bottling up the feelings. Some specific tips and exercises will help to resolve the issue and problems.

If you want to discuss some issues or problems, then pick a neutral time to time. Timing plays a vital part in the relationships. Dull time means that when you both are calm and relax. A problematic conversation will only go well when you both are ready to deal with it.

State and tell the problem shortly and briefly. Get on the point, and explain how it does affect you. Cut out the unnecessary details.

Avoid the blame game. The blaming and pointing out the mistakes of your partner will make him/her defensive and emotionally distant. It only will make things complicated.

Show Empathy More

Other than sharing your feelings and desires, it is essential to understand your partner. Try to see the situation and interpret it according to the perspective of your partner. Empathize with your partner. To do this, you have to put your thinking and perspective sideline.

To minimize the conflicts, you and your partner need to share the feelings often and take them supportively and constructively. This approach promotes the sense of safety even in the times of vulnerable and personal conversations.

Whenever you need to do a difficult discussion, you need to prepare yourself to forgive and open up to compassion. For constructive results, you must talk to your partner with a strong intent of understanding him or her.

Always try to be a haven for your partner. Partners need to feel safe with each other to make the relationship successful. It can only take place when you try to focus on one partner at a time. When one partner is explaining the problem, then others should listen and understand it.

When your partner sees that you are listening and understanding it, then he/she will be less defensive and will able to tell you everything that is bugging him/her. Listen without interrupting your partner.

Try to stay on the same topic while discussing a difficult question. It is easy to jump from one topic to another and from example to the example but do not do it. It will lead to issues, and your partner will not be able to answer them coherently. When the subject tends to shift continuously, then problems are not usually solved.

Respect is a vital element of every relationship. Always be respectful to your partner when both are going through heated discussions. Work on your anger issues. Being angry and exploding on your partner will erode your relationship. Seek therapy to cope up with your anger issues.

Be More Forgiving

Every relationship faces hard times. There always comes the point when one of the partners ends up hurting the other. It can happen in anger or in out of ignorance. Sometimes misunderstanding also becomes the reason for fights.

Feeling hurt is excruciating and is very difficult for people who have attachment-related anxiety. They tend to think that they are unworthy of love and are flawed. They flood their minds with sad and depressing.

It leads to self-criticism and makes the relationship destructive. When the person is hurt, he/she tends to recollect the bitter memories. If you are related to this, then let go of the past and learn to forgive. By adopting the habit of forgiveness, you will overcome the anger that is hurting your heart and soul.

This not only implies to your partner, but you should also be there for your partner as well. It is not essential to have a perfect balance, but being comfortable with the balance you have is vital. If you want your needs and desires to be fulfilled, then be expressive.

But if the circumstances are bitter and suffocating and you decide you leave, then formulate a plan that will help you to walk away. There is some recommendation that will help you in this matter.

Construct a support system. Breakups are painful, and you eventually need someone to lean on and share your profound and sad feelings. Share your honest opinions and struggles with close people, so they completely understand you and support you when deciding to end your relationship.

One of the most challenging parts while leaving a relationship is that you need someone else to rely on and support you other than your partner. You use to count on your partner to lean on and for emotional support, but now you need new people. Having a support system will help to comfort you and will provide you with a secure and safe base.

It is okay to feel unhappy and even cry when you feel like it. When you lose an essential person in your life, it is natural to feel sad and lonely. Do not push your feeling under the rug. It is terrible for you and will affect your mental health. Mourn and give yourself time. Time heals everything. There will be a time if that person will no longer matter to you.

You keep reminding yourself that you are a valuable person. Always remember your strength and power. This can seem challenging to do in times of misery and sadness. Consider and pay attention to what your friends and family like and appreciate about you. They interact and socialize with you because they want you and like you.

Choose the right and healthy ways of coping with your stress and sadness. When you are going through a problematic hard time, it is always an excellent option to take care of yourself. Make yourself busy with your favorite activities. You might want to go shopping, eat your favorite food, or have sex. Then go for it. If doing such activities makes you less stressed, then do them right away.

You have to be smart and considerate about them. You can make the situation worse by buying Porsche or eating a lot of unhealthy food. Take part in the activities that will make you happy in longer terms. Eat healthy and fresh. Walk and exercise daily. Sleep and wake up the appropriate time. Perform spiritual rituals to cope up with negative thoughts and energy.

Do some meaningful work. Doing meaningful work brings a sense of engagement, which is a beautiful cure when you feel disconnected. Volunteering work at shelters and schools bring a feeling of comfort and peace. Gardening is also beneficial in such cases. Helping others brings a sense of having value and connection. You feel happy and relaxed when you help others.

You should be prepared to go back to your partner. There are probabilities that, at some point in your life, you will think about the idea of going back to your partner. The good times will appear in your mind, and you will think about the mistake as well. You might also think about doing things differently and better this time.

Before picking his calls or meeting him again, think about the difficult time you've faced while living with him. Remind yourself why you left him. Talk to your supportive friend and discuss the situation. Finally, when you conclude that leaving him was the right decision, remind yourself that this weak moment will pass.

Forgive yourself if you try to go back to your partner. There are times when you feel sad and lonely; then you try to reach your old partner. You will see yourself in the arms of your partner before you realize what you've done. When you realize your mistake, then put an end to it. Everyone goes through weak moments, so try to forgive yourself.

Hopefully, this has provided you with the guiding light to reshape your relationship. By making minor changes in your habits, you can create a path towards a healthy and happy relationship. Compassion and understanding each other is key to a successful relationship.

Consult a Professional

The information provided might not be enough for you. Maybe you still not able to cut off the patterns of the anxious attachment. In this scenario, consider couples therapy. If you are the one showing the toxic behavior, then go for individual therapy.

Develop a secure base with your therapist so that you can share everything. Your therapist will guide you and assist you in cutting off the problematic behaviors and negative self-perceptions. Find a therapist with whom you can emotionally connect because there will be many heartfelt discussions that can only be done with the person you feel connected and safe.

CHAPTER 2 - How to Decode Cryptic Messages?

Like it or not, most communication nowadays is done through words – either written or oral. With the internet, writtencommunication through email or chat messages becomes the
norm, which means that your ability to read people should not be limited to just face-to-face conversations. Often dubbed as reading between the lines of reading the room, it is important for you to distinguish between what people SAY and what they MEAN.

A word of caution before we go any further: you should know that there are people who mean just what they say. The NT types are usually the ones who will tell you exactly what they want, and it would be in the most literal way possible—although, of course, this may vary depending on the situation and the unique style of the person. In theseinstances, I want you to follow a rule in law: when the words are clear, you interpret them as straightforward and apply accordingly. Only when it is ambiguous and vague should you consider the other cues indeciphering exactly what a person is trying to say.

Being a Better Listener

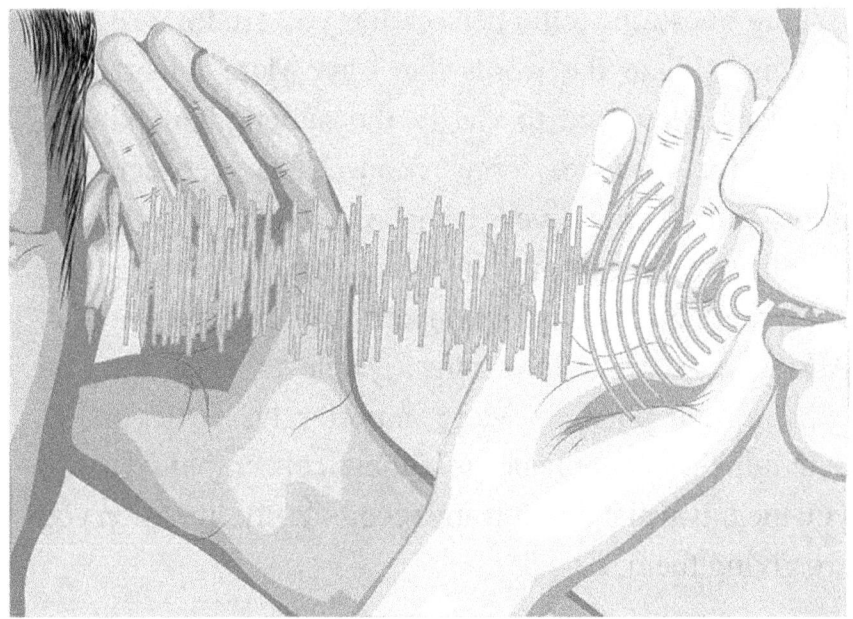

The first step in learning how to read between the lines is listening with as much attention as you can muster. When listening, your main goal should be to learn new information. Do not be one of those people who simply listen to be polite to the person talking. Instead, aim to find out something or glean information from them. You need to be curious about what the other person is saying; otherwise, you won't absorb anything. Here's a test: if you walked out of a conversation without learning anything new, then you weren't listening.

How do you become a better listener? Here are some tips:

Ask More Questions

Asking questions tell a person that you are interested in and listening to the words they say. More importantly, questions allow you to clarify the situation, making it easier for you to forge connections between the information being given. It makes it possible for you to simplify the image in your head, arrive at conclusions, and practice empathy or sympathy, as the case may be. Asking questions allows other people to elaborate and explain their position. More importantly, it encourages truthfulness in people because they feel compelled to tell you the unvarnished truth and recognize the attention you are giving them.

Practice Active Listening

This is a technique that has been used for years and can help you understand and create a story in your head. According to the director of the Center for Leadership at Northwestern University, active listening is simply repeating back what the speaker just said to you. It is like a little recap just to make sure that the two of you are on the same page. The fact is that while listening, there are lots of opportunities to misunderstand what the other person is saying. Active listening or a recap of what the other person said tells them that you are on the same page or if not, it lets them correct any misconceptions you might have about the situation.

Wait Before Responding

Except for the instances when you need clarification, it is important to stay quiet until the speaker is through. It is a typical rule in debates, meetings, and conversations, but you'll be surprised at how often people fail to follow this basic rule. The fact is that people can be so impatient that they do not even bother listening to a proposal completely before deciding to voice their thoughts, opinions, arguments, or even agreements. It can be frustrating for the speaker and makes it impossible for you to fully absorb all the ideas at once. Also note that every interruption can distort the message the person conveys, therefore making it more difficult for them to explain their standpoint.

Take Note of the Tone

A low voice adds a sense of authority, a high-pitched one conveys nervousness, stammering can indicate doubt, and fast-paced words can indicate anxiety. Also, paying attention to which words are given emphasis can change how the sentence is perceived. For example, they may be emphasizing the word maybe, or perhaps they stuttered the word yes as a reply. It could indicate that although they want to say NO, they are put in a position where they can't refuse.

Take Note of the Modifying Words

During your first few years in school, you are taught about sentence structure. There are the subject and the verb. I ran. I walked. I ate. These are all complete sentences, and they're as straightforward as they come. Even with those words, however, you can quickly say something about the talker in that all of those things were done in the past. After all, all the verbs are used in the past tense.

Most sentences are not that simple. When speaking or writing, people use adjectives or adverbs. They use modifiers that lengthen the sentence while at the same time, adding a bit more information on the activity and the speaker. The modifiers or added information in those sentences are quick and fast food. They're little clues that tell people more about what you are trying to say.

For example, quickly can imply several things depending on the situation. It could mean that a person is late, which is why they started to walk quickly. It could mean that they're trying to catch the bus or even arrive home ahead of someone. It tells you that there is something more to the story than simply walking towards a specific goal. The defining words fast food could indicate that a person did not have the time to cook or that they are still hungry.

Take a Holistic View

Reading between the lines effectively often means looking at the whole picture. You watch out for the words, the tone, the facial expression, and the gestures a person makes to fully understand what they're trying to tell beneath the surface. There will be times when the message is confusing as what a person says is the opposite of what their body is saying.

So how do you make the call? How do you decide between these two messages?

If you want to play it safe, then sticking to what a person is saying is almost always the better option. You listen to what they say, and you interpret it without considering the subtle body language that indicates the opposite. However, if you are confident of your reading and know the person fairly well to take that leap of chance, then do so! Just keep in mind that your actions have consequences, not just with yourself but with this other person.

Follow Where the Line Leads

You'll also notice that many people ask seemingly polite questions that lead them to the information they want. It is fairly common in first dates when you want to find out about sensitive information through seemingly simple questions.

Here are the typical statements that, when combined with the tone and body language, can mean completely different things:

- I do not kiss up to anybody – I do not care what people think; I am going to say what I want to say.

- I do not care what anyone thinks – I am insecure and worry about what other people might think of me.

- It is not you; it is me – It is you that is the problem.

- I have to learn for myself – I want to be independent, or I do not want you to see me be stupid.

- I am just crazy like that – I have no idea what I am doing, and I want people to find it amusing.

- What do you do for a living? – Usually, this is a polite way of asking a person how much money they're making. It isa need that connects with socio-economic security.

- We need to talk about our relationship – This can be a dangerous thing when said by a woman. Usually, this statement is said when a woman wants to reassess a relationship or tell her partner everything she thinks is being badly done in the relationship.

  Deep down, he's a good person – Everything this person has been doing so far indicates he's a bad person.

- Do I look fat in this? – I know I look fat, but I want you to tell me otherwise.

- I am always honest; if you do not like the truth, then do not ask me – I do not care if what I say will hurt your feelings; I am going to say it anyway.

- Fine, let's talk – If this comes from a man, this is usually a sign of resignation. They're willing to talk, but they're not going to be happy about it.
- Do you think she's pretty? – If this comes from a woman, this can be her asking if you are too stupid to admit that you find someone else prettier than her.

- It is nice meeting you – I probably won't remember yourname later.

- Nothing – If this comes from a woman, this can indicateanger or frustration.

I want you to remember that these interpretations aren't 100% accurate. The translations vary depending on the situation and the person you are talking to.

CHAPTER 3 - How to Stop Blaming or Insulting Each Other, Making Accusations, Losing Control of One's Emotions, Sometimes Starting to

Scream or Swear

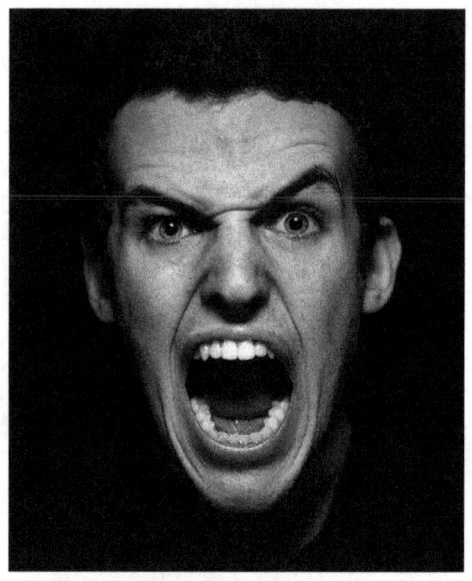

There are several ways to communicate with your spouse without offending their feelings or increasing arguments. One can remain assertive and put their point across in a more non- offensive and effective manner by using a series of highly proven communication tactics. Though communication styles can vary, the ultimate goal should convey your point more convincingly and persuasively to avoid hurting the other person's feelings and to prevent any potential misunderstandings.

Here are some tips that will help you avoid fights or communicate without getting offensive.

Know the Other Person's Perspective

Almost always, there are two sides to every story. Likewise, any disagreement has two distinct angles. It can simply be a matter of perspective. Your partner may be seeing things differently from you, and unless you are open to hearing their perspective, you won't know what they are thinking or how they see things. Listen, and understand their perspective rather than staunchly believing that yours is the only right way of thinking.

Show genuine interest in understanding them even though you may not necessarily agree with them. Many times, we may not agree with what our spouse says or believes. However, it does not mean we should not lend them a patient hearing or understand where they are coming from.

Control Your Verbal and Non-Verbal Body Language

Be cautious with your honestly and straightforwardness at times. You want to be truthful and communicate your feelings, yes. However, truth should also be accompanied by compassion and kindness. Do not take potshots at their dreams or ideas. Even if you think something is not going to work, tell them kindlier. For example, your spouse may develop a business plan that you know is not feasible in reality. Keep your words and actions in check.

Instead of making fun of the plan of their ideas, sit with them, and talk to them about how it can be much better if they put in some time, effort, and thought into it. You want to be honest rather than mislead them, but you also want to do in a manner that is not hurtful. Do not grimace or use offensive/derogatory words. Never get personal or rake up past issues in the present argument.

Construct Your Sentences as Opinions and Not Facts

When you tell your spouse something that can be potentially offensive or hurtful, do not put it across as the ultimate gospel truth or fact! Facts work for people who have a more open and liberal perspective. However, it may seem accusatory or similar to personal attacks for people who are not open to understanding a different perspective. Do not force your perspective as the only truth. Avoid criticizing, demonizing, or condemning people.

Instead of using statements such as you are wrong, try something like, I think you may not be right there. You are stating it as a perspective or opinion instead of brandishing judgments. You can also agree with their justification or perspective if the two are consistent. It reveals that your statement is not directly addressed to them in a hateful manner or to get back to them. Avoid exaggerating reality. Do not use words such as never or always. In the heat of the moment, we use idioms and phrases that stretch the truth. Do not resort to hype roles; stick to honesty. Do not allow your emotions to speed up.

Do Not Take Disagreements Personally

Being honest and being right are two different things. You can be wrong and honest for all, you know. Just because someone is stating their point honestly, does not make them right. Similarly, you can be right, honest, and end up hurting your spouse's feelings. Be genuine about your perspective, but if your spouse disagrees with it, do not take it personally. There may be a perspective or justification for their disagreement.

Resist the urge to transform their perspective to match yours. Just listen and absorb what they are trying to communicate. They have the right to their opinion and honesty just as you had a right to yours. Value your opinion, point of view, and perspective. Even if you do not disagree verbally or vociferously, remember your opinion is valid. You have as much right to be honest about your perspective as the other person.

If you offer an honest perspective, and your spouse is not open to hearing from you, pushing the issue will only worsen and create hurtful feelings. He or she may not be ready to agree with you. Avoid succumbing to the temptation of getting the other person to agree with everything you are saying. Sometimes, people should be allowed to make mistakes. Also, if they do not agree with you, it does not make you wrong. It just means the person has a different perspective, which you should not take too personally.

Tips for Diffusing Arguments with Your Partner

Arguments are an inescapable part of married life. If a couple says they never argue about anything, chances are they are lying. When two distinct individuals are involved, there are bound to be differences. There are heated discussions with people we truly care about or those we are close to. It is naturally true for our spouse too. Arguments may not be avoidable. However, not letting things snowball or get bigger is completely within our realm of control.

Pick Your Battles

In a perfect world, all arguments will end with both parties agreeing to each other's perspective and moving away in a fulfilled and positive manner. However, the reality is far different than the perfect couple kingdom we dream of building. Differences do not automatically evaporate in thin air. The key to conflict management is learning to identify a lost cause. Pick your battles wisely. Know when it is not going to be worth it to put up a good fight.

Look at the overall good rather than holding on to your viewpoint in a stubborn manner. If budging slightly will save you time and plenty of heartaches, it may be worth it.

Understand that there are topics where differences will always exist. It is sensible to avoid these topics.

Calm Down

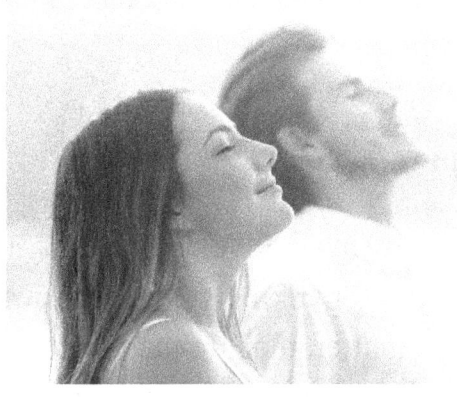

Even minor arguments can snowball into large issues if they aren't tackled or nipped in the bud. If both you and your spouse let a minor issue blow up into something huge by letting your emotions get the better of you, there's going to be nothing but fights. Damaging wordscan cause irreparable damage to the relationship, which you or your spouse may later regret. Avoid letting your emotions get the better of you in any situation and stay as calm as possible.

Practice anger management hacks such as deep breathing or countingup to 20. Take a break from the argument if you think it is on the verge of becoming more intense. Go for a walk, give it some time, andcome back with a fresh perspective. Avoid all this by being calm. Each time you find your anger rising, do something relaxing, therapeutic, and stress-busting before going back into the discussion. It won't just reduce your anger but also give you greater clarity of perspective. Sometimes, when you give it time, you'll realize that you hadn't seen it from the other person's point of view.

Stick Only to the Topic

A healthy argument is always to the point and non-personal. There's no place for raking up past issues or hitting below the belt on matters that are unconnected or irrelevant to the topic of argument. If you use personal insults or hit the other person's character, it reveals a lot about yours. When we are seething with rage, it is easy to lose perspective or broaden the scope of our fight. The dispute or difference becomes a scope to settle scores or get even with your partner by using various attacks.

This annoyance invariably includes all topics under the sun, including unfortunate personal attacks, making matters worse. For example, you may start fighting that it is always you who is doing all household chores, while your partner watches television or plays virtual games. It does not mean you can tell him or her about how everyone in their family is lazy, low on ambition, and good for nothing. They may, in return, be shocked about how you are belittling their family and may say it to you.

To which, you will go on to reply that exactly six days, an hour and 36 seconds ago, he or she had said demeaning things about your family too. What you are doing is using a real current issue (not contributing towards household chores) for settling earlier scores. It does not resolve your current issue and makes past grudges even worse. Do not use a small argument about doing the laundry as a full-blown excuse for lashing out at your better half's character.

Watch Your Body Language, Tone, and Mannerisms

Hurtful and destructive confrontations comprise a bunch of painful and hurting insults that are hurled back and forth. Shouting at the top of your voice, displaying aggressiveness through body language, keeping a more standoffish stance, raising your tone, and more are all signs of harshness. Sometimes, even without noticing or knowing if we come across as highly hostile.

Of course, you can see yourself in the mirror; otherwise, you'll know how hostile you look. Sometimes, while talking, a person will slowly raise their tone unknowingly and demonstrate their rage-filled feelings!

Speak in a gentler, calm, polite, and neutral manner. It will make you come across as more assertive, and people will listen to you. Rather than screaming and yelling, talk to people in a more assertive, calm, and confident tone. Irrespective of the nature of the discussion, keeping a friendly disposition and attitude will ensure that the conflict does not escalate.

Accept Your Differences

In an ideal world, all arguments will end with both partners settling their differences and agreeing with each other's perspective and walking away into the sunset holding hands. Reality and expectations are diverse worlds, though. For god's sake, you are a couple, not a pair of Siamese twins. Have you ever wondered how boring life will be if your spouse is exactly like you? There will be differences. However, these differences are the basis of making your relationship more exciting.

It is a good complement when you and your spouse combine forces to create a stellar relationship. Spouses needn't always think or be alike. Their differences can be a good complement to each other. Married life and communication become easier once you accept that there will be differences, and consciously work on these differences.

CHAPTER 4 - Managing Problems and Negotiating Solutions

No two people can live in the same household day-in, day-out, for years, without learning how to compromise and negotiate.

Negotiation is not always possible, but compromise should never be one-sided. The goals should never be that of deprivation or sacrifice, but one of providing for the needs and wants of both in various ways that are fair and balanced. An alpha partner should never strive to always get their way. Neither should the more beta partner give in an excessive amount. Both hardline positions have their problems.

What's the Difference in Negotiation and Compromise?

Compromise is a process of agreeing to give something up to reach a common point of agreement between two parties or individuals. A good compromise is made in a positive light and for the benefit of the entire situation. It is the right way to handle some situations in which you and your partner find yourself at odds, but not too far apart. One example is if you both want to go out to dinner but can't seem to agree on the time. You want to go earlier to get home and watch a movie that's on at a specific time. Your partner wants to go later because they hate driving through heavy traffic. You can come to a compromise by leaving slightly later to avoid the worst of the traffic and set the DVR to make sure the movie is recorded in case you are late getting back home.

Negotiation is a bit different. It is used to incorporate a little compromise and leveraging to get exactly what you want and a little more when the gap is much larger between acceptable terms. One example of this is if when planning to go and meet with friends, your partner says they can't stand being around X and Y, but Z is okay. You tell them X is coming along, but you can invite two of your friends to help distract you from your dislike of Y. In this negotiation, you are both able to hang out with your preferred friends at the same time, and everyone is a winner.

Why Both Are Needed Skills in a Successful Relationship

You will have times that come around where strong compromise and negotiation skills are required to keep the peace. Not everyone will be on the same page at all times. Whether it is due to a lack of common interest, personality clashes with friends, difficult relationships with vital family members, situations will arise that necessitate negotiation. It is not bad skills to learn for life anyway. It can be used in almost any circumstance, including dealing with other friends, family, co-workers, and more.

Compromise Should Involve Both Sides Giving to Meetin the Middle

Compromise in a relationship should always be fair and balanced. Both sides should be willing and able to give something to achieve a final objective. The compromise should also be made positively. You should always strive to not let any person sacrifice what they feel is important to achieve this peace. It is done in a fair, equitable, and balanced way.

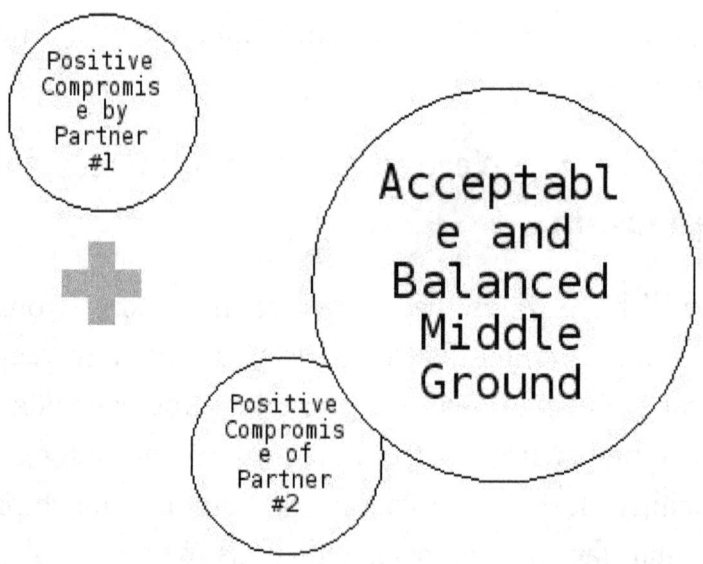

In the above example of a compromise in leaving to go to dinner, time was found that allowed the partner concerned with heavy traffic to go at a less busy time, and the partner concerned with missing the movie could rest at ease with it being recorded if they failed to return by the time it started. Neither one sacrificed anything to achieve a balanced solution.

Negotiation Is a Higher-Level Way to Get What You Both Want

The art of negotiation takes more time and planning to get the desired result, but anyone can learn to master it well with their partner. You will begin to think about possible negotiation scenarios as you get more comfortable with their likes and dislikes versus your own. It is impossible to live a life of relationship bliss without knowing how to both compromise and negotiate for resolutions.

Never Discuss Compromise or Negotiation When Angry

Things never go well when try and reach a compromise or negotiate when one or both partners are angry. It is hard for everyone to get past emotions and focus on a real solution. Take some time and let anger pass before attempting to negotiate any type of compromise. It is difficult when it involves tough subjects like dealing with ex-spouses or family gatherings when the family dislikes your partner. Solutions are possible, but all details have to be considered.

Involve a Mediator if You Get Stuck

If the situation seems hopeless and you cannot seem to get past the problem and find a solution, locate a good mediator to assist. You canuse the help of a mediation service or ask an impartial friend or relative to help you sort things out. It is vital to ensure you use someone that won't slant things in either individual's favor. It also should be someone that is not prone to gossip. Try and keep any disagreements you have between the two of you.

CHAPTER 5 - Insecurity

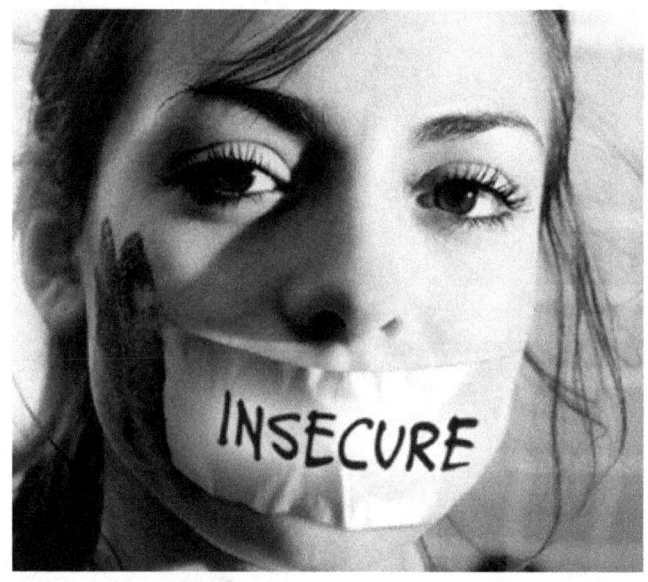

Symptoms of Insecurity and How to Recognize Them

Blaming

If you are always reprimanding or blaming your partner for everything, you need a rude awakening. This happens when your ego is controlling your relationship and utilizing manipulative tactics to do it. Do you ever assume responsibility for the things that you do? Would you be able to move to one side and think from another perspective without accusing the other person? The
ego will want you to find fault and scrutinize for others' mistakes. It will do everything and anything to

transfer blame and criticize another person. Shockingly, that thing we evade is generally what we end up receiving in our relationships.

If you fail to take responsibility for yourself, your ego will help you project all this onto your partner.

Playing the Victim

Are you playing the unfortunate victim card in your relationship? Do you always compare yourself with your partner? Is it true that you are continually putting yourself down? An unhealthy ego will help you reinforce negative actions as opposed to positive ones. It will cause you to focus too much on your imperfections. If you are doing this, it is unquestionably time to venture back and conduct a recheck on your relationship. You are not a saint.

The time has come to be responsible for what you are bringing to the table and stop constantly blaming your partner for everything.

Being Jealous

Jealousy is the green-eyed monster, and it usually sets the stage for negative drama in a relationship. Ego tends to feed on self-esteem and the absence of acknowledgment. A cherishing relationship depends on the regard and consciousness of each other. Love does not contribute to comparing, putting down, and criticizing as ego does. It is a show that turns into the most astounding type of negative drama in any relationship. If you are in an abusive relationship, your ego won't let you leave because of jealousy. What is making you consider these ideas? Does your partner make you question the validity of your relationship? It means you need to venture back and be straightforward about identifying the abuse in the relationship.

Fearing Rejection

This kind of dread prevents you from proceeding onward and accomplishing any of your goals. When you stop yourself as a result of this dread, you are unfair to your relationship. Changing the way you perceive things as oppose to being disabled by the anxiety and uneasiness caused by your ego will be a healthy way to increase self-esteem. Negative self-talk will only feed your ego. Do not compromise on who you indeed are to surrender to your partner's ego. This is anything but healthy. A loving relationship depends on mutual respect and acknowledgment. On the off chance that you are feeling rejected, maybe it is time to re-evaluate your relationship.

Always Having the Last Word

Your ego has a way of making every little thing about you and turning it into a one-person play. If you find that you talk a lot about yourself and do not ask about your partner, well, you are immensely ego-driven. The ego assumes a superb role in shielding us from accomplishing total harmony and joy. It is the mind's method for controlling. It will likewise create situations in your account that do not exist. If you find that you need to have the last say in all things, it is time that you venture back and discovers the root of this need. Do you feel like you are better than others or the second rate? Do you lack self-confidence and, in this manner, need to demonstrate that you are worthy despite all the trouble? The ego will make you conceal your sense of mediocrity by overhyping yourself. If you and your partner quarrel a lot, your ego probably fuels these fights. Is this how you feel necessary in your relationship?

It is essential to take a step back and observe your relationship at times. You need to identify when you are the one in the wrong and making mistakes. Take a look at your actions and acknowledge when they are driven by ego. You have to let go of your ego if you want a robust and healthy relationship with your partner.

So, if you have a big ego or your love is egotistical, what should you do?

For the narcissist, being correct all the time is deeply connected with their sense of self-worth. In this way, the individuals who can't relinquish their egos do and say anything they want, and they always think they are correct. Tragically, this will be at the expense of a lot of other things. Their need to always be correct can cost them their relationship with colleagues, supervisors, kin, relatives, and their partners. Sooner or later, you have to understand that the bogus self-esteem you get from adhering to your ego and being correct does not exceed genuine happiness.

Being true to yourself and practicing mindfulness will enable you to understand that you can't be right in every circumstance. There will be certain situations where you make a mistake, you have a wrong mentality, or you are mostly on the wrong side.

It may be hard to admit this at times; however, having the ability to concede when you are wrong can be quite liberating. Assume responsibility for your actions and decisions, and you will soon see that the ball will be in your court!

You do not have to be better or higher than everyone around you. The need to be this way can be quite destructive for you. A great sense of ego leads you to believe that you are superior to every other person. It is similar to remember that you do not need to be correct always. Understand that you do not have to be better than everybody else, either. That is not a healthy level of competitiveness in anyone.

There will always be somebody better, prettier, more astute, quicker, wealthier than you. No matter how old you are, this will always be the way of things.

Rather than contending with others along these lines, why not consider improving yourself? You are entirely unique. Focus on how you can improve yourself, and every one of your relationships will take a turn for the better.

Exercise: It is imperative to see how activity impacts the body as well as the mind too. Daily use is essential in the individual life. At the point when you practice regularly, your account discharges endorphins into your circulatory system, which improves your mind-set. Also, your psyche is occupied from your restless musings. Practicing has been deductively to help your general state of mind and decrease the indications of nervousness and sadness. As physical exercise increments, so improves your anxiety. A few activities to take an interest in that have been explicitly connected to tension are yoga and judo. This is because these activities for an individual to be careful in their developments and center while clearing their brain. These synthetic concoctions that are provided in mind are appeared to diminish melancholy and uneasiness fundamentally. Training supports confidence, improves certainty, enables you to start to feel engaged and reliable, and causes you to manufacture solid and new social connections and companionship.

Begin a healthy diet: The mind requires an enormous measure of vitality and sustenance to work effectively. Healthy nutrition can bring enormous changes in your physical health. A terrible eating regimen implies that you are not providing the supplements that are required for your mind's synapses to work effectively. In light of that, it might be worsening the manifestations of your nervousness. By eating a sound eating regimen and filling your plate with entire and new nourishment, drinking the perfect measure of water, and guaranteeing that you are taking in the correct nutrients, minerals, and trans fats day by day, you are giving your cerebrum the proper nourishment to capacity and battle anxiety. A solid eating routine likewise implies dealing with your gut and stomach related tract. Recollect that a sound eating routine removes improved beverages like frosted teas, soft drinks, and prepared natural product juices. Studies have demonstrated that individuals who drink over the top measure of pop each day are over 30% bound to experience the ill effects of nervousness and melancholy than those who do not. Unsweetened beverages like plain espresso, homegrown teas, and water with the organic product in it area far more beneficial alternative when keeping your body and cerebrum hydrated. Caffeine is likewise a supporter of tension side effects and ought to be curtailed to battle the symptoms of caffeine.

No more liquor: liquor is a focal sensory system depressant and is a known reason for tension as we all know that it is very harmful to ourhealth. A few people do attempt to dull the impacts of their nervousness by drinking liquor; however, actually, alcohol is regularly the base of your tension. Liquor intrudes on rest, gets dried out the body, and occupies an individual from managing the current issues instead of going up against and recognizing the root and reason for their anxiety.

Catch up on your rest: Bad dozing propensities affect an individual'sstate of mind. It is because the mind's synapses need time to rest andrecharge to keep the body's mind-set steady. Legitimate, eternal rest enables the cerebrum to adjust hormone levels and allows an individual to all the more likely to adapt to their anxiety. Unfortunate dozing propensities and sleep deprivation needn't bother with synthetic compounds to be amended. Awful resting propensities canbe rectified utilizing standard techniques including melatonin, teas, homegrown mixes, exercise, and contemplation. When you ensure that you are getting high, quality rest, your mind will start to address its hormone levels.

Begin to address your feelings: This covers dealing with your negative contemplations and frames of mind broadly, and being restless miracles the body's hormones and powers the brain to create more synthetic concoctions to attempt to feel upbeat. In the end, the cerebrum gets exhausted and can't deliver the hormones expected to battle sickness and tension. Via preparing your psyche to consider reflection emphatically and care thoroughly, you can change your recognition on what's going on and start to assume responsibility for your negative considerations. By battling and hushing your very own negative contemplations, you can work through your nervousness, ensuring that you are better ready to recuperate in your relationship. Make sure to rehearse all types of positive confirmation, which incorporates excusing yourself, appreciation for your life, and consideration to other people. When you can get positive, uneasiness begins to slow, and you are better ready to speak with your accomplice without negative, foolish conduct subverting you. Continuously recollect that you are responsible for your own life. If there are circumstances that are making your tension erupt, you can transform them.

CHAPTER 6 - Spiritual Healing Techniques

As a person who has been cheated on, what happened is degrading and unacceptable. You will find yourself asking why, and you might even blame yourself for it. You might think that
you are not good enough and that you do not deserve to be loved. This pain shall go on, and memories of that painful experience will keep coming back to you if you do not move on. You will only be able to forget the pain if you allow yourself to heal, and you will only be able to save your relationship if you allow yourself to forgive.

It will be easier for you to heal from betrayal if you avoid bringing back the past. First, it will just cause old wounds to open up again; and second, it may cause a misunderstanding between you and your partner. You've surely fought enough when you first found out about his infidelity; bringing back these memories after a long time might get back these old fights. Most importantly, you won't be able to take one step forward and leave it all behind if you keep reminding yourself of what happened in the past. Even though it is something that should not be forgotten, you must not bring it back over and over again for new memories to take its place.

Eventually, it will become a lesson for you and your partner and a mistake that must not be done yet.

As a lesson that you and your partner must've learned by now, remember to keep an open line of communication between the two of you because you must've realized by now how vital communication is in a relationship. Always talk things through no matter how nasty the situation gets because it is through talking to each other, you will understand the cause of the problem and its probable solutions.

Lastly, if you want to heal, then do not be paranoid. This may be a tough thing to do, mainly because you have already experienced being cheated on, but it is something that you must strive for if you want to move on. Even if it's hard, you must learn how to trust your partner again. They say trust is earned and not given, so the better thing to do is exert willingness to trust your partner again. Give him room to improve and to prove himself. Do not be too paranoid of all his actions—believe that he will not do it again and take his word for it.

Trying to forget such a painful phase in your life is very difficult, but surely you can do it! It just takes a lot of courage and willingness, and eventually, you'll find yourself looking back at something that once caused you pain but has now made you stronger and wiser.

How to Regain Your Partner's Trust

This is dedicated to the one who has made a mistake of betraying their partner. Restoring your partner's faith is not an easy task; you must know that you're in for a challenging journey. But remember that this journey may be full of challenges, and there will be times that you will feel like giving up, but what's more important is the prize at the end, and that is a strengthened relationship with your partner.

First things first—if you wish to regain your partner's trust, then the first thing that you must do is to take full responsibility for your mistakes. Do not go, "I did it because you did this and that!" on your partner, it will only make things worse. Remember that the decision to commit infidelity came from you and you alone, you could've suppressed it, but you did not. However, take this as a lesson and own up to your mistakes. Show your partner that you are deeply sorry for what happened and that you realize what evil you have done.

After owning up to your mistakes, the step is for you to apologize and promise never to do it again. Say the sincerest apology that you could ever muster and mean every word of it. However, a mere excuse is not enough. The more critical part of this apology is the promise that you will not commit the same mistake again. At first, your partner might doubt your words, but if you show her that you meant what you said and that you are living up to your promise, then there should be no doubt that your partner will trust you again. It will take a lot of work, but as long as you meant everything you said, then your hard work will surely reap positive results. You must keep in mind if you wish to regain your partner's trust is to be completely honest with your feelings. Do not keep things from your partner anymore, most especially if it concerns your relationship. Lying to your partner won't do you any good. If your partner observes that you are completely honest with her again, she will learn to trust you again, and she will also eventually start opening up to you again. Maintain this culture of honesty within your relationship, and this will inevitably lead to the return of trust between you and your spouse.

Love and Long-term Relationship

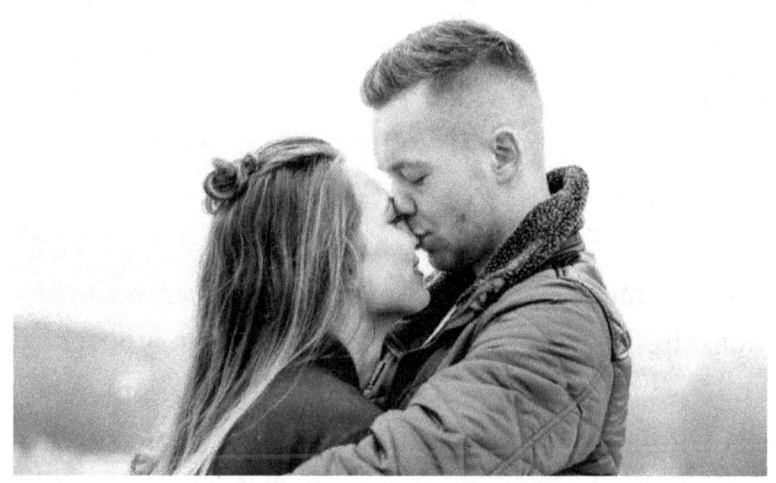

To tend to a relationship that has been bruised by betrayal, pain, and distrust is difficult and takes a lot of sacrifice, understanding, and determination. Instances of infidelity in a relationship are something that can be easily shrugged off. It is the worst thing that could happen to two lovers. However, if both sides agree to settle their differences, let go of the pain of the past, and move forward together, they will definitely develop a strengthened relationship filled with lessons from the past. The continued existence of a love relationship, satisfying and exciting to both partners in the post-affair marriage, is no accident. It involves becoming aware of your needs, of what you want in your relationship, and of letting your spouse know in a caring way. It requires that you let him know what statements and actions hurt your feelings or make you angry. Loving again also includes being sensitive to your partner's needs and encouraging him to express them. Finally, it means accepting your spouse for what he is, an imperfect human being like yourself.

Rebuilding trust	Follow-through
	Avoid Emotional Triggers
	Communicate!
	Be realistic
	Take your time

Embracing self-forgiveness	
The ways to proactively buildtrust in your relationship.	Awareness of your partner's emotion Turning toward the emotion Tolerance of two different viewpoints Try to understand your partnerResponding with empathy
The tasks of the betrayed	Ask questions that help you understand the meaning and the motives
The tasks of the unfaithful	Freely admitting fault Fully accepting responsibilities Humbly asking for

	forgiveness Immediately changing behavior

CHAPTER 7 - How To Stop Negative Thinking In Your Relationship

Are We Both Willing to Change Our Habits?

There is one widespread problem that comes from resolving our frustrations with our spouse's habits. When someone denies that the habit is bad at all, it leaves their partner feeling
frustrated while simultaneously cutting off any possibility of resolution.

In dialectic behavior therapy, we must consider our spouse's frustrations as valid if we want to have any hope of resolving the problem. It is another issue of whether you want to be right or loved.

You may believe your habit is acceptable, and even if you completely do not understand why your partner would think otherwise, you need to accept the fact that they are truly upset about it. Your spouse is not "wrong" for feeling the way they do.

Recall our lesson about the importance of subjectivity in communication in a relationship. Everyone thinks they are right. This is a very human thing. We believe that our partner is crazy for not agreeing with us, in the same way, we think that all the people who do not share all our views on significant issues must be crazy.

You just must keep in mind that other people do not all think the same way; they all think they are just as right as you do. Any time you are trying to act like you are better than your spouse for not having the habits they have, try to keep in mind that there are things you do that bother them. It is not the habits themselves that are the core issue, although you can both work on those habits. The core issue is learning how to be more tolerant of what your spouse does, even if it annoys you.

They see your habits to be just as annoying as you see theirs. To fix this situation, it is not the habits that need to change as much as it is your attitude. All of us are human, and we all do weird things because we are not perfect.

This is the kind of issue that challenges marriages. Be forgiving of each other's annoying habits instead of being mad at them for not changing.

How Do We Work Together to Strengthen OurRelationship?

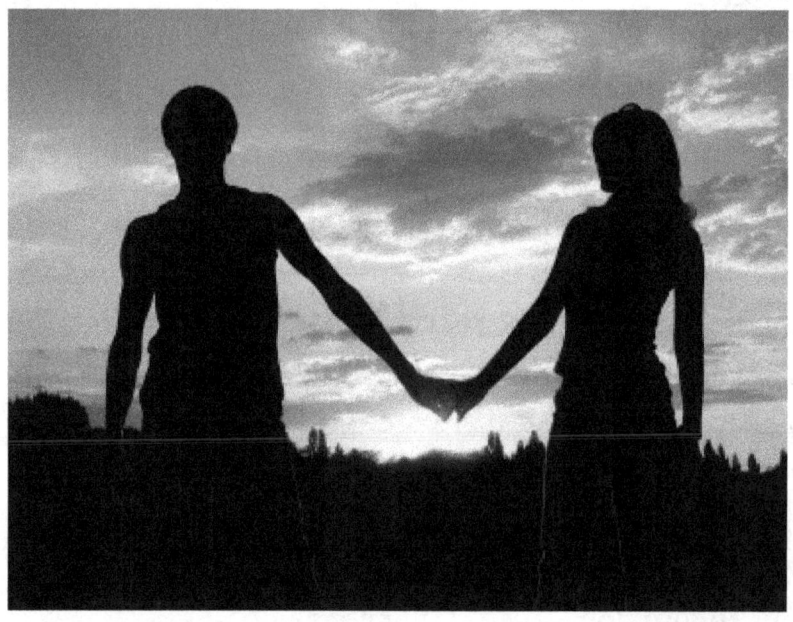

Besides the last question, this second-to-last one depends on the moston the quality communication you had with your spouse for every other problem. You cannot make yourself a better, healthier couple before confronting all the more significant issues we addressed.

Armed with the emotional understanding you have now, it is up to thetwo of you to figure out how you will work together. How will you ensure the problems you had the last time you tried to make up will not come up again? What will you do in the future if you run into this disagreement again?

The answer to the first question at least has something you can fall back on. If the two of you find that the same problems come up again—even ones that you thought you worked through in here—you should read back through it and see what insights you can find here. As much as I believe in the insights written below the dialectical behavior therapy questions, I am referring to the insights you get from each other.

What is more important than anything you read in these pages is what you say to each other in your conversations. Even the topics of the discussion can go by the wayside if you are learning how to have productive, open conversations.

Any relationship problem can be resolved if both people in the couple know how to have this kind of conversation. It is a conversation where both can say whatever they want without having to be afraid.

They must not worry anymore because they know the foundations of their marriage are strong enough to work through anything that comes their way.

You can have this kind of conversation in your marriage even if you still do not feel like you have had it up to this point. This was written for people who did not already know how to do this. It starts from the beginning with the most basic ideas of communication, and this kind of open conversation is the natural progression of that.

Where Are We Headed as a Couple? Where Will We Be in 5 Years?

This question is highly intertwined with the one when you see your spouse as a crucial part of your life. Think past yourself and think about you, your spouse, and your household.

For the last question, I asked you to hold off on thinking about the two of you as a unit for the extent of the problem. I wanted you to think only about yourself and where you might end up.

Do not see this question as totally separate from the last one. Instead, ask yourself how the future you imagined for yourself as an individual fit into this future with your spouse and family.

One of the reasons you hesitated to get a divorce (if the extent of your relationship issues is this serious) was because you envisioned this future together. It is a tough thing to let go of. There is no one else you can share this exact future with. Ask yourself if fighting for this future is worth it.

At the same time, do not let the enormous life shift that a divorce would become the thing that prevents you from getting it. If a divorce is what you as a couple need, then you should agree and go through with it.

But it is not likely that this is the case since you are nearly at the end of our relationship. If you did not have any hope that your relationship could get better, then you would not have come this far. So, you should take this opportunity to figure out what kind of future the two of you imagine for each other.

Start by telling your spouse what future you imagine them having. Then take turns. Enjoy what they say your future will be like. Figure out how both of those individual futures work together to keep a household.

It can be easy to think of ways that your spouse might get in the way of the fantastic future you see for yourself but try to look at it in a more positive light. Having someone to support you no matter what you choose to do is a real benefit, even if they will sometimes get on your nerves.

It should not take a long to figure out what you need to do. If you want to have a future together, then talk about what that future will be. Do not let yourselves delay it any longer with your hesitations about what might come.

We might as well have someone with us to be there no matter what happens, even if we wish they were not there sometimes. It is better this way than to leave it all behind, except, of course, in the case of an abusive relationship, but that would be a topic for another.

When you plan a future with your spouse, this is where things can start to get sappy. And that is OK. Just do not expect this to be the lifeblood of the marriage, because this will not be the thing that lasts.

The thing that lasts will be the commitment you make to each other as you show through your actions. You can show each other why you are there for them every day with all the little things you do. Any time you do something for your spouse, even something minimal, you remind them that the two of you are in this together.

From now on, you can look beyond just this aspect of it. Not only are they going to be with you, but they will be with you for as long as you imagine a future together.

Therefore, it is so beneficial for the two of you to envision this future together. If you have this same vision in your heads, you both feel like you have something you are striving for when you try to keep your relationship thriving no matter what happens.

You may regret things you say to each other or do or do not do. This is entirely normal, even in the healthiest, most conscious relationships. But if you both have an idea in our head about where you want your lives to go, you will be able to survive anything that life or your spouse throws at you.

Since you have both put in the work up to this, it means you want to be together, too. Do not underestimate the importance of that. When two people are willing to be together despite all they have been through, that is a powerful thing.

What Now?

The final question is no longer about what you will do to work together in general. You must both face your vices and strengths and make up your mind on what you will do now in this specific situation.

At first, you do not want to go back to the questions you already answered, unless they call to you. When you reach this last question, your mind should already be formulating something about what you will do.

When you come to one decision together, bring everything you have learned into it, remembering the mistakes you made before, so you do not make them again. They say maintaining a healthy marriage is a 24/7 job, and it is not just a cliché.

Do not expect everything to be perfect from this point—instead, use the tools you have been given to settle the problem.

Not everything can be summarized that has been covered in here. However, you could say the teachings come down to a few things: (1) the idea of dialectical behavior therapy, that is, teaching couples how to focus on one issue at a time instead of having wandering conversations that do not stick to anyone issue or resolve anything, (2) productive communication, which is all of the ideas of voicing your thoughts while also being receptive to ideas your spouse tells you, (3) problem-solving, the skills revolving around looking at the issue for what it is and making attempts to fix it.

There is much more than this, but if you feel overwhelmed after going through it all and needing something to sum it all up to make it easier to re-read, this would be a decent way to compile it all into a few bullet points.

It is both of your choices that you want to do from here. You might think you have gotten everything you need out of this, and you just want to put it away for a while and see how you do without it. It will still be here for you if you should ever need it.

There was one final note I wanted to give you, and it is that both of you should get into the practice of trying to look at your relationship from an outside perspective. You will never be able to do it entirely, but the mere attempt will get you to see things more clearly.

CHAPTER 8 - Moving on With Your Life

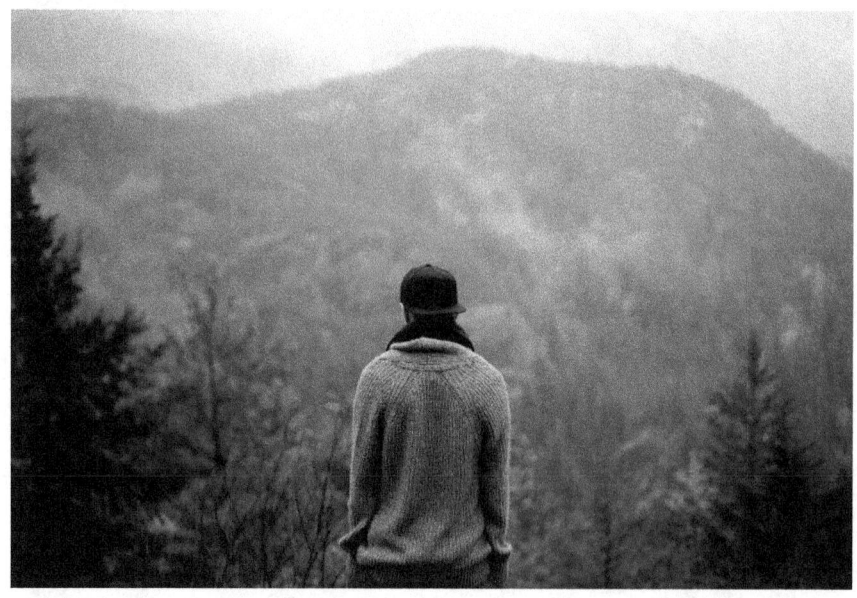

When you come out of a codependent relationship, often, your confidence can be at an all-time low, and you may find that you have lost a lot of yourself that was formerly tied up
in your relationship identity. Now is the time to re-discover who you are as an individual and firm up your needs and desires. You need to be gentle with yourself and start rebuilding your confidence. Codependents are so caught up in what it means to be a couple, only focusing on the identity of their relationship and not on their identities, that once you leave a codependent relationship, you may struggle at first to find your feet in this strange new world as a singleton. This is a

common side effect of a codependent relationship. Be kind to yourself as you discover your new identity as an individual and not part of a couple. Take time to find your wants and needs- based upon your personal feelings. Understandably, some people find it hard to establish their desires. Still, I have included below some strategies to help you move forward and rebuild your self-confidence, allowing you to make choices and decisions based on what you want. Building your self-confidence and self-esteem begins with learning to love yourself and wholeheartedly accepting yourself for all that you are.

Rebuilding Your Self-Confidence

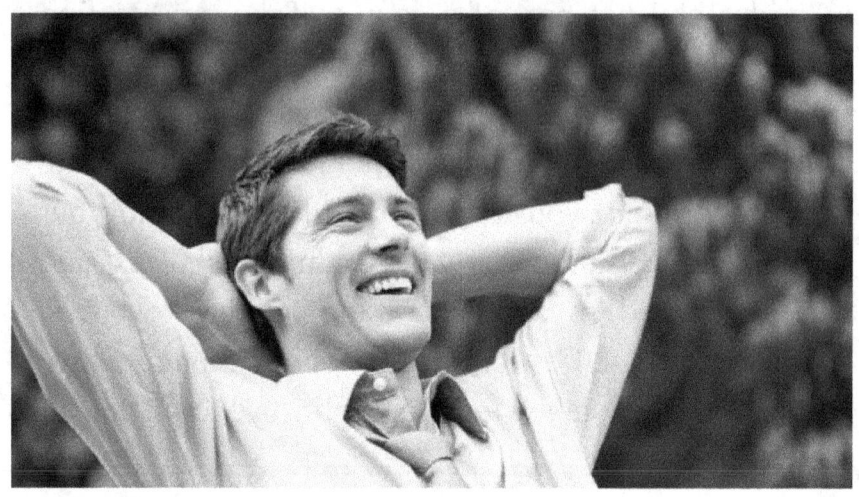

Stay away from negativity and negative people

Negative people can harm your self-esteem and self-confidence. You want to stay away from people that bring you down and constantly challenge your actions. In a healthy friendship, two people pull each other up when they feel the other is not doing something right, but negative people often challenge others for entirely different reasons. Try and limit your contact with these kinds of people.

Develop a Positive Attitude.

You are starting a new stage of your life, so try and develop a new positive attitude. Often, we listen to that negative voice in our heads. When you hear yourself saying something negative or derogatory, try to turn it around and come back with something positive.

Likewise, when you put off doing something new or that will take you outside of your comfort zone, try and approach the situation without prejudice and pre-emptive assumptions, instead flip it on its head and approach new problems with an open mind.

Accept Failure

We all fail at some point in our lives. Instead of seeing failure as a bad thing, try to reframe it positively. Failure is not bad, and it only defines you if you let it.

Pick yourself up and continue. Accept that there are just some things in life that are out of our control, take what you can from experience and learn from it. The faster you accept failure, the easier you will find it to move on to better things.

Accept Compliments

Most people are genuinely nice. If someone offers you a compliment, try and resist the urge to disagree with them; instead, teach yourself to simply say thank you. People do not go out of their way to be demeaning; remember that they wanted you to feel good about yourself.

Compliment Yourself

Compliment yourself every day. Try and find something you did well, or something complimentary about the way you look, for example, 'That jacket looks very flattering on me,' or 'I worked hard on that project yesterday.' Learning to love yourself is essential to your overall well-being. Take responsibility for your feelings and acknowledge them.

Coming out of a codependent relationship can be a steep learning curve. Understanding that you are only responsible for your own emotions and not the feelings of other people is a hard concept to understand. But you need to learn how to take care of you and let others determine what is right for them. You are not responsible for everything that happens in the world, nor anyone else's reaction to it. Just remember that you are too busy taking care of your emotional health to interfere in anyone else's.

Do Not Compare Yourself to Others

As Teddy Roosevelt once said, "comparison is the thief of joy." You are unique. There is only one of you in the world, so why compare your unique individuality to others? Stop concentrating on other people and begin to focus on being the best version of yourself that you can be. Comparing yourself to others takes the focus away from the most important person, which is you. Stop wasting your time measuring yourself by other people's standards and start making your way in the world.

Let Go of The Past

Everything we go through in life, every situation we encounter, makes us who we are today. Instead of shutting the past away in a box at the back of your head, let yourself feel the emotions connected with the past. Feel them—do not suppress these emotions, and then let them go. You are not who you were yesterday, and you won't be the same person tomorrow. Understand that you will tie yourself to negative experiences from the past by not dealing with these emotions. It is OK to cry or feel angry about past experiences. Stop playing the victim. Decide to let past hurts go. Accept responsibility for your part in the situation and stop blaming others. Journal if you think it will help. Keep the focus on the present.

Practice Good Self-care

This is the ultimate way to express self-love. Ensure you are getting everything you need; the right foods, enough sleep, some exercise, connecting with others, and the world around you, and engaging in activities that will expand your personal development.

Believe in Yourself

Who will believe in you if you do not first believe in yourself? Trust that you can do anything you set your mind to. After all, you managed to disengage from a codependent relationship and put down the framework for rebuilding your life. Stop listening to negative people, remember past successes and achievements, and recall them every time you hear that voice saying you can't do something. Turn the sentence around. Instead of saying, "I can't," try saying "I am working on…" Self-doubt is a big destroyer of self-confidence, and the more you give in to it, the greedier it will become until it drags you down, and you stop believing in yourself at all.

Learning to Love Again

At some point in the future, there will come a time where you feel ready to start again and open yourself up to the possibility of having another intimate relationship. However, if you found healing from a codependent relationship challenging, the thought of entering into a new relationship can appear terrifying. Breaking away from codependency does not mean not getting into a relationship ever again or becoming a relationship phobic. Instead, it means that you can take your time to find a relationship that is right for you.

Avoid jumping straight into another relationship. If you have just left a codependent relationship and dive straight into a new romance, without first taking some time to heal and rebuild your emotional health from the ground up, you will find yourself sucked back into the compulsive-obsessive cycle of codependency.

When considering entering into a new relationship, think objectively and neutrally about your fundamental reason to be with someone new. Do you feel the need to play rescuer? Are you struggling with your new identity or feel like you have no validation if you are not in a relationship? Are you simply in love with the idea of being in love? These can be ample warning signs that you are not yet ready and need to do more work to not slip back into old behaviors.

If you do find yourself in a new relationship for all the wrong reasons, you need to take a step back and perhaps, re-read the parts on ending and healing from a codependent relationship and begin to take care of yourself before thinking about committing to another potentially damaging connection that could wreck all the good work that you have done. However, if you feel that you have put enough distance between yourself and your past codependent behaviors, and you feel confident that you are ready to start again, here are some simple ideas for taking that first step into a healthy, mutually beneficial relationship.

Try and visualize yourself in a new relationship that meets all of your needs

What does your new relationship look like, and how do you maintain the feeling of a connected, loving relationship without needing to take over responsibility for the other person or their actions? Partners in a healthy relationship do not need to spend all their time together; they are happy for the other to spend time independent of them. In a healthy relationship, neither partner is responsible for the emotional well-being of the other, and this can be achieved without being cold or disconnected. You can bond with another person without taking on their needs as a duty that you must perform. Your obligation is first and foremost to your own emotional, physical, and mental well-being.

Do not let Fear of Ending up in Another Codependent Relationship Put You Off

You have new tools to recognize a codependent relationship; you can establish why you want to start again with someone new. Companionship? Mutual interests? These are great reasons for being in a relationship. Trust that you have not only managed to free yourself from codependency, but you have the toolkit to help you avoid being dragged back into that damaging cycle once again.

Define Boundaries from the Start

This time, you know what a healthy relationship should look like. This should help you set new positive relationship standards. Keep reinforcing to yourself that you won't associate with anyone who mistreats you or relies excessively on you for his/her needs. Remember why the past relationship ended and identify early signs that predict a similar pattern.

Be Open to New People.

Learn to identify positive and nurturing relationships from negative and destructive ones. Spend time with balanced people who accept you unconditionally for who you are, not what they want you to be. Let down your guard and stay open to new people, but stay away from people who display highly obsessive-compulsive traits or addiction dominated behavioral patterns.

CHAPTER 9 - Getting to Know the True You: Being Your Authentic Self

Do You Know Your True Value?

Many of us look down on ourselves, and we fail to give ourselves the credit that we deserve. We might indeed have gone through experiences that may now affect the way that
we look at ourselves. We might have gone through a lot of hurt and abuse and even a very challenging childhood. But these circumstances do not have to continue to define you and hide the unique qualities that make up the real you.

Reasons Why You Are Unique

Just in case you are not convinced about how unique you are, here are some significant reasons proved by science why you should start seeing yourself differently.

- **Your unique genetic composition is the only one there is and will ever be**: Research has shown that humans are somewhere between 90 -99% different genetically. Such a big difference, is not it? This is to say no one is exactly like you genetically (even if you have an identical twin), and no one can ever be like you no matter how hard they try. Why try to compare yourself with or even become someone else when there is only one of you in existence? You simply can't be them, and they can't be you.

- **Your personality is unique:** A person's unique personality is made up of their temperament, thoughts, attitude, behavior, character, and beliefs. No two people will have the same combination of these qualities at every given time. Your personality is how people see you and how they often try to describe you—meticulous, quiet, outgoing, selfless, funny, proud, humble, loud—these are all components of a person's personality, and yours is a unique one.

- **Your experiences are unique**: Your entire life experiences, as well as your day-to-day experiences, are what make you an extraordinary person. There are no two people who have had the same experience throughout their whole lives. Even if you live together, work simultaneously, maintain the same schedule, you will find that your point of view of these experiences differs. So, your life experiences are unique to you.

- **Your purpose is unique:** You should believe that you have aunique purpose in this world. You do not have to live the lifethat someone else has lived. You do not have to be your fatheror your mother—you should be yourself instead. Even if you follow in their same footsteps, you will still find that you cannot produce the same achievements, something will differfrom the other, and this difference speaks of the uniqueness of your life and who you are. You have such a unique purpose in life; therefore, you should pursue it and embrace it and not live someone else's life.

Building an Unbeatable Self Confidence That Will Always Defeat Jealousy

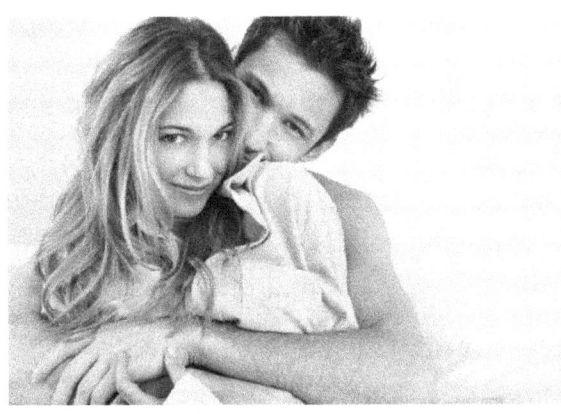

Self-confidence is very important when talking about jealousy because a reduced self-confidence can bring about jealous feelings. If you suffer from low confidence, then you are bound to get jealous at some point.

- **Self-confidence can be learned:** Some people have described themselves as not being confident naturally. They have stuck to that belief from childhood, causing problems with jealousy and the likes in their relationship and life in general. The truth is that even if you are genetically inclined to be withdrawn and shy, that does not mean you should have low self-confidence. You can learn to be confident in yourself gradually, and in time you will see the changes confidence can make to your entire life. There are so many people today that were initially not confident in themselves but have grown from that stage into living their dreams and achieving their goals with high confidence.

- **There are no losers, only winners**: Never see yourself as a failure or a loser at anything you do even if it does not work out a hundred times. Life is not a competition, and there are no losers. You are a winner if you choose to see yourself that way and behave like that as well.
- **Life is a process, and you can get there as well**: So, you are not where you feel you are supposed to be, so what? And you have tried and failed so many times. We have all failed at something as well, so you are not alone. Some people can't cope with failure, and others can't stand the fact that those they consider their mates are getting ahead of them in life, so they turn these feelings to jealousy and anger. You need to understand that life involves a process, and the fact that you have failed ten times does not mean that you cannot succeed on the eleventh try. Also, the fact that you feel you are behind in life does not mean that you cannot reach where you want to be eventually. There are a thousand and one examples of people who have made it great in life but failed initially.

- **There is room for everyone to shine:** Just like the moon and the sun, they shine their light differently, and they do not compete with each other because they know their uniqueness. That is how you should see the world. No one is taking your opportunity or your job. If you did not get that dream job and someone else got it, you should believe that the job perhaps was not for you, and you can get another opportunity. Do not imagine the competition and become jealous when someone like that makes a pass at your partner. There is room for everyone to shine our lights as brightly as we desire.

- **Start loving yourself:** It is surprising how some people can love a partner so much and show themselves no love at all.

  You should start loving the person that you are and treat yourself better. Do things for yourself and be selfish sometimes—it will make you feel great. Treat yourself to something special on occasion. Something that is just for you—a nice spa, an expensive meal, a new dress, anything that screams 'treat!' Start doing things, not for others but yourself as well, and you will notice how good it makes you feel. You do not have to wait for someone to say those words to you so you can feel good about yourself. Learn to start loving your unique self and see the boost in confidence that it will bring.

- **Stop doubting your abilities**: The worst thing you can do to your confidence is to question yourself. People will doubt you at least until you can prove them wrong, but when you start doubting your abilities, then there might not be an opportunity to prove anyone right or wrong. Even if no one believes in you, you should still believe in yourself—that is how a lot of people have kept going until they succeeded—by believing in themselves. Whatever it is that you want to embark on, you need to tell yourself that you can. The more you keep feeding your mind with a positive thought, the more your confidence will improve, and you will get better at whatever you try. You can't depend on what people say to give you the confidence you need; you need to be the first and only coach of your life.

- **Start doing what you used to love:** Are there activities you used to love doing but have lost interest in because of how your life has changed? A great way to revive that confidence is to return to some of the things you loved doing, like playing a sport or a musical instrument, fishing, skating, singing, dancing, traveling. Whatever it is, start again if it makes you happy—even if you weren't so good at it, this could be an opportunity to get better and do what you love.

- **Try out new interests:** Perhaps you have been passing by a dance school and wondering what it would look like if you enrolled in a class. Or you have recently been interested in playing a musical instrument and have held yourself back because of what your partner or friends might say. You should take that positive step now and try out one or two interests you have nursed for a long time. It is never too late to try out something new—unless you are physically limited. So how about trying something, and if you like it, then continue doing it—you will see that your confidence continues to grow as you make such bold steps.

- **Work on you continuously:** Working on yourself is very important to building a high self-confidence. These are areas that you can start improving. For instance, if you haven't felt confident about your body and have always been threatened when someone with a great body makes a pass at your partner, then why not decide to achieve that great body that you want as well? Remember that you will be doing this for yourself and not for anyone else—it is to make you feel great and confident again. So hit the gym and start working hard to achieve that great body that you want. Perhaps it is something about your appearance or your language that kills your confidence. You can learn how to improve these things as long as it makes you feel more confident. Go get it!

- **Re-assess your company:** One cause of low confidence without even knowing it is the kind of company that you keep. Do your friends look down on you or tell you that you are not good enough for a role or something you want to try? Do you have friends that laugh or mock you when you fail at something? These are confidence killers, and you should avoid them as soon as possible. Great friends should be able to encourage you to reach your dreams and not kill your confidence. So, what kind of things do you hear from your friends? Does it help you grow your confidence? If it does not, then you are better off without them. You should stick with friends that are confident and do not see you as a threat to their progress as well. Friends who are secure in themselves and can inspire that in you as well are friends indeed.

- **Take good care of yourself:** Just like I said about loving yourself, you can't love something you do not care for, so start taking care of yourself. Scientists have shown that taking good care of you can reflect in your overall demeanor and confidence. Pay attention to your hygiene. Take showers regularly, put on clean and appropriate clothing, apply pleasant scents, and pay attention to your hair care. Take care of your living space as well, and keep it clean and tidy.

- **Strive to be a better version of you:** Make it a habit of taking regular appraisals of yourself. Where are you now, and who do you want to be in one year or five years? Always strive to improve yourself and keep becoming a better version of yourself. Remember that it's not about becoming someone else or competing, but it is all about yourself and building a secure and confident you!

CONCLUSION

Emotional codependency is a product of childhood trauma and emptiness that was built on the day you promoted to adulthood. You have suffered enough all these years as you grew up, abandoning yourself for the happiness of others and never caring about your own needs. But this has to stop and it has to stop now. You are an individual with the same right to live as anyone else in the world.

Your opinions and expressions matter as well and you are allowed to reject anything you don't feel connected with. Saying no to codependency, anxiety and all the problems related to your relationship means saying yes to life!

Good luck!

CPSIA information can be obtained
at www.ICGtesting.com
Printed in the USA
BVHW090333040521
606332BV00006B/1076

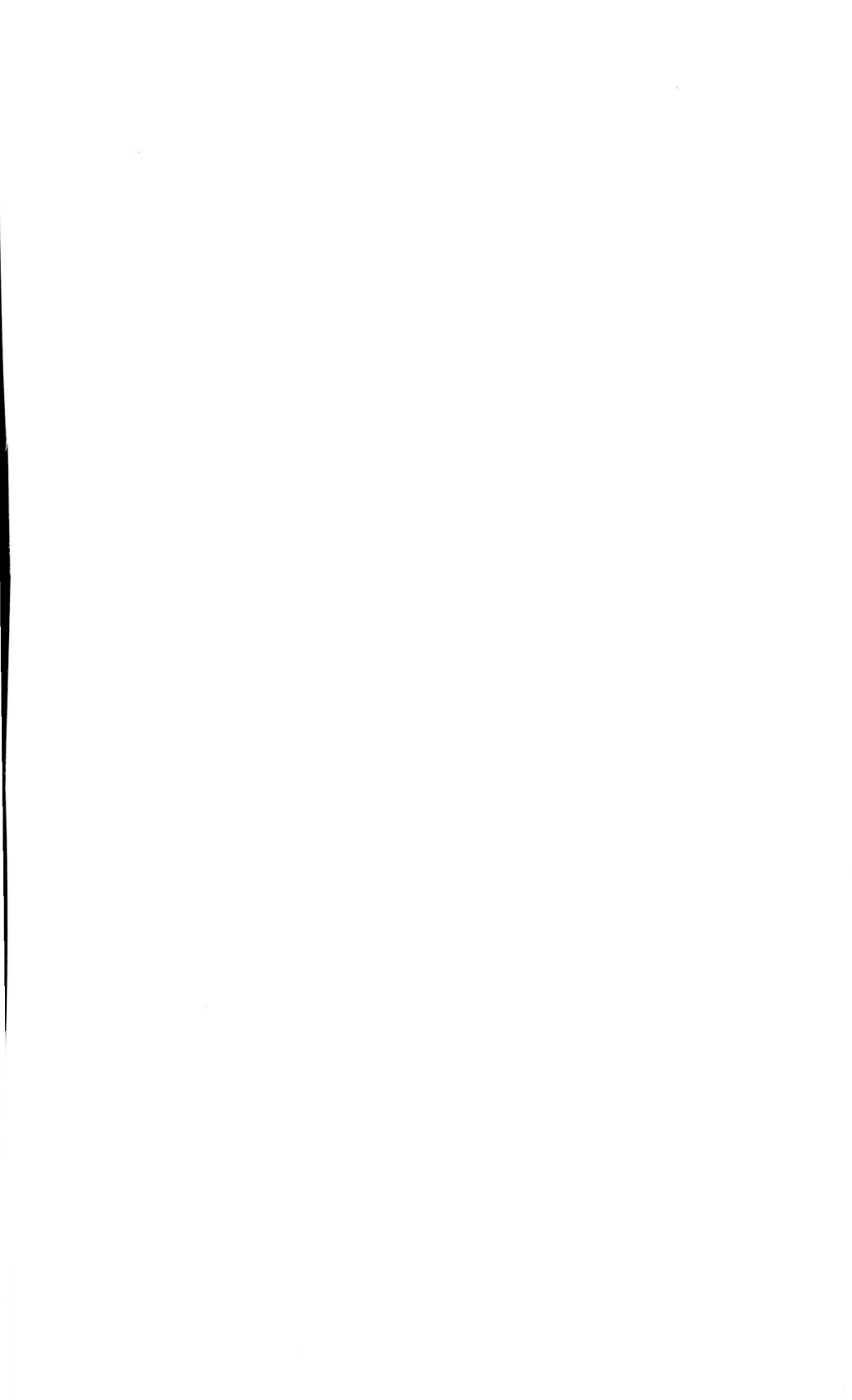